I0439438

The TRUTH about S.T.D.'s

Tony Davis,P.H.T.
(Perfect Health Teacher)
DID YOU KNOW THAT ALL S.T.D.'s ARE LIES?
NOW YOU DO AND I'M GONNA PROVE IT TO YOU!

Copyright © 2014 by Tony Davis
All rights reserved ISBN 978-1495396700
No part of this book may be reproduced,stored in a retrieval system or transmitted in any form or by any means:electronic,mechanical,photocopying,recording or otherwise without the written permission of the author of this book: Tony Davis

Warning:This book is protected by the United States Government at www.copyright.gov

To order additional copies of this breakthrough book, please go to www.amazon.com They are $10 each.

NOTE: All the sayings in my book were invented by me unless otherwise specified. Also,certain names have been changed to protect people's privacy.

For free updates of this book please visit:
www.happyforever.us

TABLE OF CONTENTS

PREFACE

We live in a world where most people are successfully brainwashed in every country in the world. There are so many stories that are 100% false but people believe them to be 100% true. Why is this happening? Because of a few reasons:

1-The stories are told over and over for a long period of time-some bullshit stories are hundreds of years old

2-People don't bother to check a story to see if it's true-they just believe it without looking behind the story for proof. Only proof makes a story true. People are gullible.

3-A lot of people are making billions of dollars telling people lies. **The more lies told=The more profit made**

The truth does hurt indeed. It hurts the profit of the evil rich greedy soulless bastards who sell people deadly products and kill them,all in the name of profit. And when I say the truth,I'm talking about this:Back in the 50's people were being lied to about cigarettes. People were told that smoking cigarettes is good for the health of your lungs when the truth is exactly the opposite: smoking cigarettes is bad for your lungs-very bad actually: it kills your lungs therefore killing you. This is just one example. There are many scams like that and in my unique book I'm gonna expose only the scams that are bad or deadly to your precious health.

DISCLAIMER

Everything I wrote in this book is strictly my opinion. However,everything I wrote in this book I based it on facts and hard scientific evidence. The information in this book is for educational purposes only. It does not constitute medical advice and should not be construed as such. I cannot guarantee the safety and effectiveness of any treatment,remedy or advice mentioned. Some of the tips may not be effective for everyone. A good medical doctor is the best judge of what medical treatment may be needed for certain conditions and diseases. I strongly recommend that in all cases you contact your personal medical doctor or health care provider before changing your diet or discontinuing any medication you are taking or before treating yourself in any way. I am not making an attempt to prescribe any medical treatment. I am not responsible in any way,shape or form for any bad consequences you might experience from taking my advice. My book is not intended to treat,prevent or cure any disease. The information provided in this book is designed to provide helpful information on the subjects discussed. This book is not meant to be used, nor should it be used, to diagnose or treat any medical condition. For diagnosis or treatment of any medical problem,consult your own physician. The publisher and author are not responsible for any specific health or allergy needs that may require medical supervision and are not liable for any damages or negative consequences from any treatment,action,application or preparation to any person reading or following the information in this book. References are provided for informational purposes only and do not constitute endorsement of any websites or other sources.

Readers should be aware that the websites listed in this book may change. This book is designed to provide information and motivation to our readers. It is sold with the understanding that the publisher is not engaged to render any type of psychological,legal or any other kind of professional advise. The content of each article is the sole expression and opinion of its author and not necessarily that of the publisher. No warranties or guarantees are expressed or implied by the publisher's choice to include any of the content in this volume. Neither the publisher nor the individual author shall be liable for any physical,psychological,emotional,financial or commercial damages, including but not limited to,special, incidental,consequential or any other damages. Our views and rights are the same:You are responsible for your own choices, actions and results. This book is presented solely for educational purposes. The author and publisher are not offering it as legal,accounting or other professional services advice. While best efforts have been used in preparing this book,the author and publisher make no representations or warranties of any kind and assume no liabilities of any kind with respect to the accuracy or completeness of the contents and specifically disclaim any implied warranties of merchantability or fitness of use for a particular purpose. Neither the author nor the publisher shall be held liable or responsible to any person or entity with respect to any loss or incidental or consequential damages caused or alleged to have been caused,directly or indirectly by the information or programs contained herein. No warranty may be created or extended by sales representatives or written sales materials. Every person is different and the advice and strategies contained herein may not be suitable for your situation. You should seek the services of a competent professional before beginning any improvement program. The story and its characters and entities are fictional. Any likeness to actual persons,either living or dead is strictly coincidental. All the information in this book is intended for general reference purposes only and is not intended to address specific medical conditions. This information is not a substitute for professional medical advice or a medical exam. Prior to participating in any exercise program or activity,you should seek the advice of your physician or other qualified health professional. No information on this book should be used to diagnose,treat,cure or prevent any medical condition. Conclusion:This book is only my opinion,my thoughts and my conclusions after 50 years of research. You and only you are responsible if you choose to do anything based on what you read in my book. Thank you very much for your acknowledgment. The author

CHAPTER ONE:The TRUTH about S.T.D.'s
Did you know that:
ALL S.T.D.'s ARE SCAMS?
Of course you didn't! Most likely you are hearing this for the first time in your entire life from me.
I know what you are thinking:how can all S.T.D.'s or Sexually Transmitted Diseases be SCAMS?
How is it possible that they don't exist? Are you shocked? Are you skeptical? Are you amazed? You shouldn't be! Life is full of surprises and in this case it is a pleasant surprise. Make that a very pleasant surprise!
You believe that S.T.D.'s are real because you have been successfully brainwashed. You,your family and your friends and the entire world have been lied to for more than 200 years. You believed all your life that S.T.D.'s are real because everybody told you so but did it ever cross your mind that there is no proof when it comes to S.T.D.'s?
Or that nobody can prove that they actually exist? I know they have some "proof" that S.T.D.'s exist but that is bullshit proof. More about that later. If you think that I believed all my life that S.T.D.'s do not exist,then you are sadly and badly mistaken!
I,too was a victim of global brainwashing meaning they washed my brain too! Meaning that they convinced me too that S.T.D.'s exist. For 25 frigging years-from 1980 to 2005-I was 100% convinced that AIDS and all the other S.T.D.'s exist even though I never really looked behind the story for proof to see if it's a true story.
"That is a mistake I'll never make"
I believed that S.T.D.'s are real all my life because that's what I was taught in high school and because everybody told me they exist.

However,back in 2005 I was on the internet looking for something and "accidentally" I saw a link that said:"AIDS is a hoax".I was shocked and curious about this link and I clicked on it immediately and read the entire website which had proof that AIDS is a scam,a lie,a hoax,a fraud,etc.

After that I found many more websites that were saying the same thing:AIDS is bullshit! Boy,did I get excited. It was one of the happiest days of my life! I remember it like it was yesterday. I believed the websites immediately because the proof they prevented was real proof and I realized that I no longer have to fear something that doesn't exist:AIDS! I also remember jumping up and down with joy because of this exciting news that changed my life forever and now it's time to change your life forever-if you are open minded,that is! Anyway,I wasn't 100% convinced that AIDS is a global deadly lie yet so I searched for even more websites,I found them,I read them and I became 99% convinced that AIDS is garbage. Then I bought a bunch of books that also told me the truth about AIDS and then I finally became 100% convinced that the mother fathers bullshitted me and the entire planet big time. After this historical discovery,I started wondering if the other S.T.D.'s are scams also. After years of scientific research I was convinced that not only AIDS doesn't exist but all S.T.D.'s don't exist either. They are all fairy tales! All S.T.D.'s are SCAMS! Do you have an "S.T.D." already or are you afraid of getting an S.T.D. in the future? You shouldn't be! How come I'm not afraid of getting any S.T.D.'s? Do I know something you don't? Of course I do! S.T.D.'s are a joke to me!

I don't fear any S.T.D.'s and I never will because I know the truth about S.T.D'.s.

Do you know what I fear? NOTHING! I don't live my life in fear like most people. There is a saying:

"A life lived in fear is a life half lived"

Before I tell you why all S.T.D.'s or Sexually Transmitted Disease are lies,first let's take a look at what they tell us S.T.D.'s are.

In case you are wondering who "they" are:

"They are your family,your friends,the people that write books and magazines,the people on the radio,the people on TV,etc"

"They=Everybody that tells you stories"

Let's take a closer look at the name "S.T.D":

STD=Sexually Transmitted Disease which according to them liars it means that you will get a disease from a diseased person if you have unprotected sex with them,right? Right my balls!

Let's start with the word "disease".

They tell us 2 things (lies) about diseases:

1-Disease are caused by germs,bacteria and viruses

2-Diseases are contagious meaning somebody that is diseased can give you their disease if you have sex with them,touch the things that they touched,be around them or touch them in any way.

Unfortunately virtually everybody on this planet believes these stories. These are true stories,right?

Fortunately,they are not! All of them are fairy tales. All of them are lies. Don't believe me? Why not? Why believe them but not me? Good question!

You don't have to believe me of course but I'm telling you that they have been lying to us for hundreds of years.

"Only one thing makes a story true and that is:Proof"

Do they have any proof? Of course not. You can't prove something that doesn't exist. But guess what? I got proof that they are liars and they have been lying to us for a very long time and are still lying to us today.

Do you find this hard to believe? I bet you do! Now,I have a surprise for you. Surprise! That's it. As long as you are alive on this planet you will experience:
"A continuous number of surprises,some pleasant and some unpleasant for as long as you live"
You might not be aware of it but it's happening to you,to me and to all of us.

It's time now folks to tell you why these 2 stories that have been fooling humanity for hundreds years,are not true. **FICTION:**

1-"Diseases are caused by germs,bacteria and viruses"

a)Germs

Germs don't make us sick. They never did and never will. Have you ever seen a germ? Has anybody that you know or don't know seen a germ?

Can anybody prove that germs make us sick? Absolutely NOT! So,we got no proof here. Are you gonna believe a story without proof? Okay,let me tell you how this global fairy tale was born that is fooling virtually everybody.

Once upon a time there was a guy who convinced an entire nation and eventually the entire world,to believe in his germ theory. His fictional germ theory caused a lot of pain,suffering and death to millions of innocent people around the world and that is still happening today.

And it will happen tomorrow,the day after tomorrow and so on until everybody finds out the truth.

This germ theory of disease was never tested under strict scientific scrutiny. This theory is bull shit. No,it's bull crap. No,it's ball shit. It's all of the above,love!
It's a very convincing global lie. This theory was even questioned and opposed from the beginning but unfortunately for humanity dissension fell on deaf ears. In other words,people who said that the theory: "Germs cause disease" is false,were ignored.
This guy's critics were never able to convince the medical establishment that he was wrong.
The "me-dick-all" establishment,which is a very lucrative business and is making billions of dollars upon billions of dollars in profit,welcomed this stupid idea of the germ theory of disease because it keeps making them a shitload of money! That's why they are full of shit!
The inventor of the incorrect "germs cause disease" theory acted by himself on his deadly mistake. He was asked by his own government to find out why drinking alcohol caused so many people to get sick. Today some of us know that alcohol is a poison with many side-effects but back then when many people still believed that demons caused diseases and science was primitive,no one knew that.
Fact:
"Alcohol is a poison that causes disease,premature aging,insanity,violent tendencies and death"
Have you ever heard the expression: "Alcohol poisoning"?
That means your body was poisoned by alcohol which is poison. Also,there is another expression about alcohol: "What's your poison"?

You will hear that only in one place or places: bars,pubs,night clubs,strip clubs or wherever they sell alcohol aka poison. Here's another secret for you: Whenever you buy alcohol at a strip club,while the strippers are stripping for your viewing pleasure,they are stripping you of your good health by poisoning you with alcohol. Also,they are stripping you of your cold hard cash. They take away your health and your money! People were pretty dumb back then. As dumb as a rock. As dumb as a rock star that is! Why are rock stars dumb you might ass? (ask!) Because they poison their body with a different poison:recreational illegal drugs. Back to the story now. So this guy went to work immediately to find out why alcohol makes people sick and he concluded incorrectly that the bacteria in the alcohol caused sickness. Not everybody agreed with him. There were quite a few smart scientists during his time who said that his theory is wrong but because the government believed this guy,any opposition to his stupid idea fell on deaf ears. What the hell are germs anyway? How exactly do they look like? Where are they exactly? Talking about germs is like talking about demons. We are talking about mythical creatures or creatures that only exist in movies or fairy tales. Long story short:
"Germs don't exist and they don't cause any disease" However,they do cause something else:billions of dollars in profit from sales of useless products that "kill"them!

b)Bacteria

Bacteria does NOT make us sick. On the contrary, bacteria is keeping us alive and bacteria is good for our bodies. Without bacteria we will all die. Did I wake you? Good! Now that you are awake check out this fact:

90% of our bodies are occupied by bacteria

Bacteria are very simple single-celled organisms. Like most of earth's simple creatures,bacteria live for two very basic purposes:food and reproduction.

They reproduce just like any other cell:through cellular division and they are responsible for eating the dead debris left behind when plants and animals die. The word usually associated with the work of bacteria is "decay." When something is dead,it decays and it is the job of bacteria to break down dead tissue at the cellular level,therefore ridding the earth of dead plants and animals. Without them,we'd be up to our eyeballs in cadavers. God bless all bacteria on this Earth-they are our friends!All bacteria are saprophytes. This is what scientists call creatures that eat dead things. Fungi,many insects,vultures and all strains of bacteria are saprophytes and are incapable of eating anything other than dead tissue like dead cells. If bacteria did make us sick,then that means they must be eating our living tissue,thus killing our cells and causing our bodies to deteriorate. But as saprophytes,bacteria cannot eat anything but dead tissue. If you are alive,then your tissue is living,therefore ,bacteria cannot harm you. At all times, you have billions of bacteria living inside of your body. Remember,cells die all of the time.

Fact:
"About 300 billion cells inside our body die daily and are replaced by new cells"

Usually,other cells are responsible for eating up these dead cells and disposing them from the body. But bacteria are also within our body to help in the elimination of dead cellular debris. We have bacteria in our throat,lungs,stomach,intestines and all throughout our bloodstream. They exist to help us digest food,they provide us with certain vitamins,they help in the absorption of minerals and they perform thousands of other functions that we need for survival. Without bacteria,our body would be overwhelmed by dead cells and we would die.

The symbiotic relationship we have with thousands of strains of bacteria is necessary for our survival,so it is ridiculous for us to think that they can cause disease. Bacteria are beneficial and vital for our health. Without bacteria we will all perish. Bacteria are so beneficial that I need to write a book about it. In fact without bacteria all animals and all plants will perish also. Without bacteria we cannot even rot after we die.

Just like germs,bacteria causes billions of dollars in profit for many greedy and evil companies.

Conclusion:

"Bacteria do exist but they do not cause any disease"

a)Viruses

You believe that viruses exist,right? Wrong! Very wrong. "Viruses never existed and they never will"

So,how can something that doesn't exist,make you sick? Let's start with the most popular and the most "deadly" virus:The HIV virus.

When people are diagnosed HIV-positive(a diagnosis that is hogwash because all HIV tests are wrong-you can't test something that doesn't exist!),the fear factor alone is enough to cause disease. The belief in viruses came about almost 40 years before the technology existed to see at the submicroscopic level using an electron microscope. Any first-year molecular biology student will tell you that electron microscopes are very poor instruments that produce black-and-white shadows of images on computer-printed electron micro-graphs that must be

interpreted by trained professionals before anyone knows what they are. When you look at an electron micro-graph, it's not like looking at a snapshot; it's like looking at black blobs on a white sheet of paper.
Unless somebody tells you what you're looking at,you have no idea what you're seeing.
Even the best trained professionals were told what to look for at one time,so who's to say they even know what they're seeing? Back in the 1940s (after over 35 years of believing that viruses must exist),a scientist manufactured the first useable transmission electron microscope:one that could see at the submicroscopic level. After studying the poor electron micro-graphs they produced,scientists finally agreed that they had found a virus. After all,the belief existed for almost 40 years;they would have looked pretty stupid if they didn't find something,right?But did they really find viruses?
Or did they just go on a modern-day witch hunt and accuse the first thing they saw of being a witch,I mean a virus? You've got to know a little something about molecular biology to really understand the existence of viruses. I'll explain what has happened,but don't worry if you don't fully understand. I doubt there's more than a dozen molecular biologists who fully understand everything they believe. Anyway, right now in your body, you have billions upon billions of cells-muscle cells,tissue cells,blood cells,bone cells and so forth. We actually have about 100 trillion cells altogether. All of these cells work together to form you. But while you can live many, many years (perhaps a lot longer than you currently believe),your cells only live for weeks or months at a time. After that,they undergo the process of cellular division. One cell splits into two cells, two into

four, four into eight, etc. Cells can only divide so many times before they get old and then they die. Their offspring can go on forever. But cells die eventually. The process is called apoptosis:a kind of cellular suicide. When this occurs to a cell,the cell dissipates inside the bloodstream and becomes a rather sloppy blob of genetic material and protein debris. Getting back to viruses,the definition for a virus is a genome wrapped in a protein sheath. A genome is nothing more than genetic material,so if a dead cell is genetic material and protein debris,then wouldn't it make sense that these materials could be misidentified on occasion as viruses?
A genome wrapped in a protein sheath is actually a dead cell or a virus. So,viruses are something dead.
Can something dead cause disease? No! Hell no. During the 1940s,scientists did not know that cells died and dissipated in the bloodstream. Instead of finding viruses,they found dead cells and their witch-hunt concluded with them believing that viruses were nonliving genomes wrapped in protein sheaths. And scientists today still believe in the existence of viruses.
Only the stupid ones of course!
There's a smart saying about stupid people:
"There is a sucker born every minute"
Just because you are a scientist,it doesn't automatically make you a smart person. Let them believe all they want but that doesn't mean viruses exist. They also tell us that viruses are invading living cells in order to force reproduction. When living cells eat dead cells (as they do all the time in the bloodstream),it could easily appear as though a virus is entering into a living cell. When living cells eat,it is known as phagocytosis. The process of phagocytosis then,has been misidentified as a virus

entering a cell. Remember that no one sees this process in live action. It must all be interpreted on a series of electron micro-graphs,which are computer-printed shadows of images on black-and-white paper. It takes experts to read these micro-graphs, and even the experts have admitted that they have mistaken dead cells for viruses on many occasions. Couldn't they have also mistaken phagocytosis for a virus entering into a living cell? I think so!

Conclusion:
Viruses do not cause disease. They don't exist.
Never did,never will.

Fact:
"Viruses=Dead cells"
Long story short: They tell us that S.T.D.'s are caused by viruses and bacteria. They are of course lying. I just proved to you that bacteria and viruses do not cause disease. And that means only one thing:

S.T.D.'s=SCAMS
Now,I would like to take a closer look at this not so deadly HIV virus and viruses. According to what they tell us,if you have unprotected sex you can get the HIV virus and if the virus is not detected in time and treated then it turns into full blown AIDS and it will kill you. Also,you can get it from "infected blood" and this deadly HIV virus has spread in every country in the world and killed millions of people and nowadays if people get infected with the HIV virus they have a chance to live longer lives or even avoid an early death thanks to the HIV pills and cocktails that are now on the market. Let's take a look at what they tell us a virus is. According to them lying vile bastards,a virus is a live microscopic microorganism that has the following bullshit characteristics:

1-It grows and multiplies only in living cells of people or animals

2-It's highly contagious and deadly and you can get it from having unprotected sex,using contaminated needles or getting a HIV infected blood transfusion

3-A virus can take over a cell and command it to multiply the virus until the cell is dead and then they move on to other cells and do the same

4-A virus can lay in wait and disguise itself

5-A virus can be dormant in the body for decades,wake up at any moment and attack you and once you get the virus it stays in your body for the rest of your life,etc

You've heard the scary lies that they have been telling us since 1980 and now it's time for me to tell you the truth. Before I do that there is something very important I have to tell you first.

Here it is:After you hear or read a story,how can you be 100% sure that the story you are about to believe to be true is actually 100% true?

How do you separate fact from fiction? I'll tell you how. You use a "secret" ingredient called proof. Do not ever believe a story 100% until you look behind the story for physical proof.

"Proof is what separates fact from fiction"

Here are 7 unique life changing breakthrough sayings about stories I proudly invented myself:

1-"A story without proof is a fairy tale"

2-"A story without proof is proof without a story"

3-"Believing a story doesn't make it true,proof does"

4-"A true story doesn't have any questions without answers and a false story has many questions without answers"

5-"A true story can be proven by anybody while a false story cannot be proven by anybody"

6-"If something exists,then it must exist somewhere"

7-"A true story is forever and and a false story is temporary"

Did it ever cross your mind that some of these "tragic" stories they tell us all the time on TV or Radio,in books,magazines,billboards,etc are actually lies? Well,guess what? They are!Surprised? You should be! All these stories about S.T.D.'s, deadly S.T.D.'s, how you get them from having unprotected sex and are a bunch of crap. Why? Where is the proof? Have you or anybody you know seen any scientific proof proving that this "deadly HIV virus" actually exists? If you find it please let me know but I'm not holding my breath because it's gonna be a very cold day in hell when you are gonna find something that doesn't exist.

I have a question for you now my S.T.D. fearing reader: What's something that you cannot hide forever? The answer is:The Truth!

"You cannot hide the truth forever"

Remember that hit TV show from the 90's that said: "The Truth is out there"? The show is fiction but the saying:"The Truth is out there" is fact. The truth is really out there,all you have to do is find it and fortunately you found it in this book. Thousands of people around the world found the truth and so did I and I am now sharing it with the world. I really care about people,I love people so much and it breaks my heart to see so many innocent people being lied to and the consequences are suffering and death. Lives are destroyed and families are ruined forever. People have been lied to enough. People have suffered enough. Millions of people are suffering and dying each year around the world and why is all this happening?

This is happening because they believe in a deadly lie, not a deadly virus. Have YOU ever see a virus with your own eyes? Can you give me the name of the asshole or the bitch who can show the world how a virus looks like? Can you tell me where I can go and see a virus with my own eyes?

Of course you can't because viruses are as real as: Superman, Spider-man, Batman,etc.

They only exist in fictional books and movies.

Fact:

"Seeing is believing"

Seeing is believing and if don't see something, then don't "be-lie-ve" it.

Fact:

"Nobody on this planet has ever seen a virus and nobody ever will"

Fact:

"The HIV virus does NOT exist"

You heard what they said which is a bunch of cruel evil deadly global lies and now it's time for you to hear the truth about what viruses really are.

WHAT VIRUSES REALLY ARE:

1-Viruses are microscopic dead genetic material,having no life at all

2-Viruses have no metabolism and they cannot process food

3-The size of a virus is so small that a cell is a billion times bigger than a virus.

4-A virus to a cell is like a fly to an elephant:How much damage can a fly do to an elephant?

5-A virus has no faculties for action of any kind

6-A virus cannot replicate itself
7-A virus cannot invade any living organism
8-A virus doesn't have any life qualities whatsoever
9-A virus is literally garbage created by the cell
10-A virus is like a dead person.
How much damage can a dead person do to you?
Guess how much proof there is that the HIV virus is a big deadly global lie? A mountain of evidence would be good,right?But no,there is no mountain of evidence here but a universe of evidence for you to examine!Is a universe of evidence enough proof for you?
The HIV virus is not in the body but in the mind.
It's all in your mind!Not literally,of course.
The "deadly" HIV virus story is garbage and it's time for you to take the garbage out!
Fact:
"AIDS is a cruel and evil deadly global HOAX"
There is literally a universe of proof that HIV/AIDS is a scam and if I give you all the proof then I would have to write a bunch of books on that subject alone!I will only give you the basic proof or enough proof.
Check out these amazing,eye opening,mind blowing,life changing,life saving facts:
1-Dr. Robert Willner was so determined to prove to the world that "AIDS" was not spread sexually or through blood contamination that in 1993 he stunned the nation of Spain by injecting himself on national TV with the blood of Pedro Tocino, a hemophiliac said to be "HIV positive".The footage was broadcast throughout Europe. Encouraged by the coverage he was receiving Dr. Robert Willner repeated his performance with many different patients in front of of the cameras of ABC and NBC.

Not surprisingly to me,this historical news was never shown on national TV or any US TV network.
Dr. Robert Willner was constantly tested and he remained HIV negative until the rest of his life.
(It is impossible to be HIV positive!)
Here are some videos of Dr.Robert Willner injecting himself with the "HIV virus" to prove to the world that he's not afraid of something that is a lie:
1-http://www.youtube.com/watch?v=26vbwILsLsY
2-http://www.youtube.com/watch?feature=endscreen&v=tQCKb1JV-4A&NR=1
3-http://www.youtube.com/watch?v=4DuEClDjZmM&feature=related

2-Dr. Paul Grinberger was given a grant from the government to study how harmful the HIV virus is and the results were very exciting for the public:
"The HIV virus is harmless,it doesn't cause AIDS and you don't get it from having unprotected sex"
Unfortunately not everybody was excited about Dr. Paul Grinberger's findings and he was fired and his laboratory shut down forever. Why? How much money will "they" be making if people knew the truth:nothing.
Dr. Paul Grinberger is a good honest man but he made the mistake of biting the hand that feeds him. It's OK anyway,because if it wasn't for honest people like him we would probably never know the truth about the HIV virus.

3-AZT began as a "cancer drug" but was withdrawn for being too toxic:like being thrown out of the Gestapo for cruelty. Its side effects include cancer,hepatitis,dementia,seizures,anxiety,impotence, leukopaenia,severe nausea,ataxia and death.

Fact:
All the people who died of "AIDS" died because they took AZT.
AZT eventually kills all those who continue to take it.
4-Over 10,000 and rising of the world's scientists and doctors are now disputing the HIV hoax,their efforts being continually suppressed by the AIDS establishment,the"name deleted"syndicate and their political and media lackeys.
5-When Germany found out the truth about the deadly HIV/AIDS scam,they got so pissed that they did this:They made a new law:
It is illegal to say that "HIV causes AIDS"This hypothesis HIV=AIDS was found ILLEGAL in Germany and the Supreme German court ruled that HIV was not proven to cause "AIDS".
6-Dr. Carlo Peschini,Specialist in Internal Medicine,Infectious and Tropical Diseases,New York:
"HIV tests are meaningless. A person can react positive even though he or she is not infected with HIV. The tests are interpreted differently in different countries,which means that a person who is positive in Africa (or Thailand) can be negative when tested in Australia. There is no justification for the fact that most people have not been informed about the serious inaccuracy of the tests. The error has catastrophic repercussions on thousands of people. Since people are reacting positive on tests that are not specific for HIV,let's please stop labeling them as 'HIV positive'"
7-A study done by Congress's Office of Technology Assessment,found that HIV tests are very inaccurate.

8-Manufacturers of Western Blot(HIV)test kit stated:
"Positive tests do not prove AIDS or pre AIDS disease status nor that these diseases will be acquired."

9-How about that? The manufacturers of the HIV tests themselves are saying that their tests do not prove HIV or AIDS. In other words the HIV tests are a waste of your precious time and money. All HIV tests that detect the "HIV virus" are bullshit. All these tests are useless and deceitful.

They do not detect the HIV virus in your body.

10-A health magazine from USA:
"Virologists have nothing new to offer. They keep coming up with excuses, they find constant growth and change in the virus structure, it evades, attacks, strange things, but none of them has the courage to explain properly how these things could possibly be so."

11-AIDS did not spread in every country in the world.
In Japan AIDS does not exist. Does that tell you something? They fooled everybody but they couldn't fool Japan. Japan has the best knowledge when it comes to health and disease and Japan is the healthiest country in the world! In fact,AIDS didn't spread to any country only the lie about AIDS spread to almost every country!

12-Even if the HIV virus existed,condoms do not stop it. If the HIV virus existed,it would be so small that it would go right through the condom and inside your body but you got nothing to worry about. Now you know the truth:HIV is just fantasy!(I love it when it rhymes)

13-Shelby Evans who has been "living with the virus" for more than 35 years:
"I have known so many people who have died of AIDS and all of them-all of them took the drugs they were told to by their doctors. I have never taken any of them and I

haven't gotten sick. Not even a cold. The doctors told me I had 5 years left to live. These drug companies that produce the deadly medication are getting very rich and people are getting very dead!Everyone I know who has been HIV positive-and that's a lot of people-has died after taking those drugs prescribed by their own doctors"

14-Professor Morton McGrath,Public Health University of Glasgow, Scottland:

"Nobody wants to look at the facts. I've sent countless letters to medical journals...they simply ignore them. The fact is,this whole HIV/AIDS story is a hoax."

15-Dr. T.C.FRY:

"We Americans are among the most brainwashed people on this planet and we always thought it was in Russia or in other countries that this dastardly practice was perpetrated. We are being lied to on a grand scale. We are unscrupulously manipulated and treated. We are unconscionably ripped off. We are pitifully ravaged in body and mind. The "name deleted" is the primary agency for originating,perpetrating and perpetuating one of the most villainous and evil scams ever concocted:The genocidal HIV/AIDS scam.

AIDS is a big farce invented and fostered,firstly,to destroy the gay rights movement and,secondly,to stake out huge new economic reserves for our (name deleted) industries. From the beginning Dr.(name deleted) and Dr. (name deleted) knew that no virus was involved in AIDS. They knew it was not contagious and they deliberately lied to the public that this "new" disease called "AIDS" originated in Haiti among the heroin users when they knew better."AIDS" was created entirely by the (name deleted).AIDS was born at (name deleted) and it made (name deleted) billions of dollars more in revenue"

16-Dr. Cathy Perris,a Nobel Laureate and Biochemist and a 1993 Nobel Prize for Chemistry:

"It's not even probable,let alone scientifically proven,that HIV causes AIDS. If there is evidence,there should be scientific documents which demonstrate that fact. There are no such documents. If there is evidence that HIV causes AIDS,there should be scientific documents which either singly or collectively demonstrate that fact,at least with a high probability. There is no such document. The HIV theory,the way it is being applied,is unfalsifiable and therefore useless as a medical hypothesis."

17-Dr. Fabrizio Alba, a specialist in infectious diseases:

"I am well convinced that the HIV virus is harmless. A major problem with the new AIDS definition is that it ignores the man-made environmental causes of immune suppression. Exposure to toxins,alcoholism,heavy drug use or heavy antibiotic use all can cause onset of the list of 'diseases' indicative of AIDS".

18-Mitch Wagner,Medical Hypnotherapist,New York:

"I have seen the constant terror, and programming to get sick and die, that people at risk for developing AIDS face. I am certain that the hypothesis that long-term drug use is primary cause of what is now called AIDS is far more likely to prove true than the failed notion that AIDS is caused by a germ. I have seen the constant terror and the programming to get sick and die. As long as we imply that 'AIDS' itself exists we are operating within the AIDS group fantasy."

19-"It was the first time a scientist had ever run away from me. Typically scientists are bulldogs. They fight for their position. But the HIV guys don't. They run."
David Rasnick on his doomed attempt to get answers on awkward questions from HIV-fantasist
Marty Berkowitz

20-Dr. Rafaelo Pagliacci:
"AIDS is a drug user's disease and it's not sexually caused or transmitted"

21-Dr. Matthew Doller:
"AIDS was always and still is a drug user's disease"

22-Dr. Chad Christmas:
"AIDS is a cruel deception that is maintained because so many people are making money from it. Take away this money and the entire system of mythology will collapse."

23-Dr. Tim Thomerson who is also a member of the National Academy of Sciences:
"If you think a virus is the cause of AIDS,do a control without it. So far it hasn't been done. The epidemiology of AIDS is a pile of anecdotal stories,selected to fit the virus/AIDS hypothesis.

24-A magazine from Italy:
"Dr. Paul Grinberger is absolutely correct in saying that no one has proven that AIDS is caused by the AIDS virus. And he is absolutely correct that the virus cultured in the laboratory is not the cause of AIDS."

25-Dr. Sergiu Nicolaescu,Bucharest,Romania:
"If there is evidence that HIV causes AIDS, there should be scientific documents which either singly or collectively demonstrate that fact, at least with a high probability. There is no such document."

26-Dr. Hans Munich,Emeritus Professor of Molecular Biology and Virology:

"The result of my intensive literature research shows that so far not one publication exists,in which is being described that HIV has been isolated,purified and characterized by the criteria of classical virology. Up to today there is actually no single scientifically really convincing evidence for the existence of HIV.
Not even once such a retrovirus has been isolated and purified by the methods of classical virology."

27-Dr. Sam Livingstone,Professor of Mathematics:

"I do not regard the causal relationship between HIV and any disease as settled. I have seen considerable evidence that highly improper statistics concerning HIV and AIDS have been passed off as science, and that top members of the scientific establishment have carelessly,if not irresponsible,joined the media in spreading misinformation about the nature of AIDS."

28-Dr. Larry Potter,Professor of Molecular and Cell Biology:

"It is not proven that AIDS is caused by HIV infection,nor is it proven that it plays no role whatever in the syndrome."

29-Dr. Rick Steinmann,Emeritus Professor of Cell Biology:

"In the old days it was required that a scientist address the possibilities of proving his hypothesis wrong as well as right. Now there's none of that in standard HIV-AIDS program with all its billions of dollars."

30-Dr. Harold Giovanni,Molecular Biologist, former editor of Bio/Technology and Nature Biotechnology:

"HIV is an ordinary retrovirus. There is nothing about this virus that is unique.

Everything that is discovered about HIV has an analogue in other retroviruses that don't cause AIDS.HIV only contains a very small piece of genetic information. There's no way it can do all these elaborate things they say it does."

31-Dr. Adolfo Ludwig,former Professor of Immunology at the University of Bern and former director Swiss Red Cross blood banks:

"The sentence of death accompanying the medical diagnosis of AIDS should be abolished."

32-Dr. Thomas Charleston,former Professor of Biochemistry,Harvard and John Hopkins Universities:

"The HIV-causes-AIDS dogma represents the grandest and perhaps the most morally destructive fraud that has ever been perpetrated on young men and women of the Western world."

33-Dr. Gil Jonah,New York Physician:

"The marketing of HIV,through press releases and statements,as a killer virus causing AIDS without the need for any other factors,has so distorted research and treatment that it may have caused thousands of people to suffer and die."

34-Dr. Adrian Baldwynn,Emeritus Professor of Pharmacology,United Kingdom :

"I think AZT was never really evaluated properly and that its efficacy has never been proved, but it's toxicity certainly is important. And I think it has killed a lot of people. Especially at the high doses.
I personally think it not worth using alone or in combination at all."

35-Dr. Emile Chateaux,Emeritus Professor of Pathology,Canada:

"Dominated by the media, by special pressure groups and by the interests of several pharmaceutical companies,the AIDS establishment efforts to control the disease lost contact with open-minded,peer-reviewed medical science since the unproven HIV/AIDS hypothesis received 100% of the research funds while all other hypotheses were ignored. How many wasted efforts,how many billions of research dollars gone in smoke... Horrible."

36-Dr. Sorensen Johanes,Professor of Preventive Medicine,NY:

"Evidence is rapidly accumulating that the original theory of HIV is not correct."

37-Dr. Brad Ford, Biology Professor:

"The cause of AIDS is multifactorial.HIV is neither necessary nor sufficient."

38-Mick Parker, former Science Editor,The Times of London:

"A kind of collective insanity over HIV and AIDS has gripped leaders of the scientific and medical profession. They have stopped behaving as scientists, and instead are working as propagandists, trying desperately to keep alive a failed theory."

39-Dr. Jason Capon,Ethicist,Head of the School of Applied Ethics,Australia:

"The orthodoxy will collapse because it flunks the practical test. The AIDS epidemic was a mirage manufactured by scientists who believed that integrity could be maintained amidst the diverting influences of big money, prestige and politics."

40-Dr. Martin Hawn, Senior Professor of Law:
"That establishment continues to doctor statistics and misrepresent the situation to keep the public convinced that a major viral pandemic is under way when the facts are otherwise. One does not need to be a scientific specialist to recognize a botched research job and a scientific establishment that is distorting the facts to maximize its funding"

41-Dr. Leo Hanks,Professor of Biophysical Chemistry,Amsterdam:
"There are many people with AIDS but without HIV, and a great many people with HIV but without AIDS. These two facets mean that HIV = AIDS is much to simple. Plausible,alternative,testable causes of impairment of the immune system which may ultimately lead to AIDS should become part of regular AIDS research."

42-Dr. Ruben Smith,Professor of Molecular and Cell Biology:
"It is not proven that AIDS is caused by HIV infection, nor is it proven that it plays no role whatever in the syndrome."
The causal role of HIV in AIDS is certainly not proven."

43-Dr. Marcus Black,New York Physician:
"The marketing of HIV,through press releases and statements,as a killer virus causing AIDS without the need for any other factors has so distorted research and treatment that it may have caused thousands of people to suffer and die."

44-Dr. Ennio Napoli, Specialist in Preventive Medicine and Infectious Diseases,Italy:
"I am not an agnostic but I am well convinced HIV is harmless."

45-Dr. Forrest Whitman,former Managing Editor of the Proceeding of the National Academy of Sciences:
"The HIV hypothesis ranks with the 'bad air' theory for malaria and the 'bacterial infection' theory of beriberi and pellagra (caused by nutritional deficiencies). It is a hoax that became a scam."

46-Dr. Liam Owens,Counseling Psychologist:
"Protecting and promoting the unproven HIV hypothesis as fact is inducing unnecessary stress,probable emotional harm and maybe even psychological murder."

47-Dr. Calvin Stevens,M.D. New York Psychiatrist:
"There is no way that AIDS can be an infectious disease. Something else must be going on. The more likely interpretation is that HIV and immune dysfunction-rather than HIV being a cause and immune dysfunction being a consequence-are both consequences of something else."

48-Dr. Bruce Barry, Emeritus Professor of Epidemiology,Scottland:
"AIDS is a behavioural disease. It is multi-factorial, brought on by several simultaneous strains on the immune system-drugs, pharmaceutical and recreational,etc. Nobody wants to look at the facts about this disease. It's the most extraordinary thing I've ever seen. I've sent countless letters to medical journals pointing out the epidemiological discrepancies and they simply ignore them. The fact is,this whole HIV/AIDS thing is a hoax."

49-A newspaperman from Greece:
"From both my literature review and my personal experience over most of the AIDS-so called AIDS centers in Africa,I can find absolutely no believable persuasive evidence that Africa is in the midst of a new epidemic of infectious immunodeficiency."

50-A magazine from England:
"They have hyped up HIV into this super-rapist but in reality the damn thing can hardly get an erection."
51-A magazine from New Zealand:
"Epidemiology is like a bikini:what is revealed is interesting;what is concealed is crucial. When AIDS patients' bodies finally break down from the effects of these anti-viral drugs,they say,'Now the virus has become resistant and the drugs have lost their effectiveness. What really is happening is the toxicity of the drugs builds up to a point where the patient cannot stand it anymore.
And of course,they say it was the virus,rather than the entirely inevitable and predictable toxicity of these damned deadly drugs."
52-Dr. Jenny Jamiesson,Professor of Pathology and Medicine:
"I stopped going to AIDS meetings several years ago. I could no longer stand the stress of restraining myself from getting up and shouting,'Rubbish!'"
53-Dr. Dimitrius Galfianakis:Professor of Mathematics,New York:
"I am suspect about everything involved in this AIDS epidemic, because if HIV causes anything,it certainly causes fund-raisers. It sells stocks. It supports dances. It sells condoms. And it keeps the AIDS establishment going."
54-Dr. Mongo Mabute :Department of Family Medicine and Primary Health Care at the Medical University of South Africa:
"The case for a link between HIV and AIDS is not proven. I would like the "orthodox" scientists to

acknowledge that in Africa there are 29 or 30 diseases which may mimic AIDS,which are related to poverty. But they will not accept that because poverty does not make them big money but HIV makes them money. If we dissidents had only one hundredth of the funds that the orthodox view has,the orthodox view would probably be dead in less than a year."

55-Dr. Aaron Delaware,Professor of Medicine:

"I have a large population of HIV + patients who have chosen not to take any anti-viral drugs. They've watched all of their friends go on the anti-viral bandwagon and die."

56-Dr. Raj Khapur:Professor of Anatomy,India:

"For all we know,it is not HIV that causes AIDS, but the so-called co-factors such as indiscriminate antibiotic use, recreational drugs,poverty,malnutrition,polluted water and pesticized food. AZT and the like (so-called triple therapy) are rank cytotoxic poisons. To give AZT to pregnant women is a crime against the mother and the baby she is making."

57-Cal Kristofferson,AIDS Activist:

"The HIV paradigm has produced nothing of value for my life and I actually believe that treatments based on the arrogant belief that HIV has proven to be the sole and sufficient cause of AIDS has hastened the deaths of many of my friends"

58-Dr. Kurt Scheimann:Virologist,Germany:

"No particle of HIV has ever been obtained pure,free of contaminants;nor has a complete piece of HIV RNA(or the transcribed DNA)ever been proved to exist."

59-At least 3 documentaries were made exposing the truth about AIDS:

a)"The other side of AIDS" by Robin Scovill

b)"House of numbers" by Brent W Leung
c)AIDS,inc by Dr.Gary Null
60-The pH Miracle Living Foundation in cooperation
with Alive & Well are 100% sure that the HIV virus
doesn't exist that they are offering a **$1,000,000** reward to
anybody who can prove scientifically in a lab that the
HIV virus exists. Here are 3 websites where you can read
about this:
**a)http://articlesofhealth.blogspot.com/2007/05/ph-
miracle-living-foundation-in.html**
**b)http://www.anderekijk.net/docs/pH_Miracle_Living
_Foundation_1M_reward.txt**
**c)http://www.blogster.com/revkenny/a-1000000-
reward-for-scientific-proof-of-hiv**
So,if you are 100% that the HIV virus exists,prove it and
you'll receive a cool $1,000,000! Keep dreaming,though.
You cannot prove something that doesn't exist,can you?
Also,many books have been written about the truth about
AIDS.Here are 30:(Is that enough for you?)
1-The great AIDS hoax by Dr.T.C.Fry
2-Fear of the invisible by Janine Roberts
3-AIDS and the doctors of Death by Alan Cantwell
Jr,MD
4-Inventing the AIDS virus by Peter H.Duesberg Ph D
5-What if everything you thought you know about AIDS
was wrong?
by Christine Maggiore
6-Positively False:Exposing the Myths Around HIV and
AIDS by Joan Shenton
7-Get All The Facts:HIV does not Cause AIDS by Dr.
Mohammed Al-Bayati, Ph.D., D.A.B.T., D.A.B.V.T.
8-The AIDS WAR:Propaganda,profiteering and genocide
from the medical-industrial complex by John Lauritsen

9-AIDS:The failure of contemporary science by Neville Hodgkinson

10-Deadly Deception by Robert E.Willner MD,PhD

11-Global AIDS: Myths & Facts by Alexander Irwin and Joyce

12-AIDS, hope, hoax and hoopla by Michael L Culbert

13-Global Responses to AIDS: Science in Emergency by Cristiana Bastos

14-Imagine Hope: AIDS and Gay Identity by Simon Watney

15-AIDS, the establishment confesses-it's a hoax by Keidi Obi Awadu

16-Good bye AIDS! Did it ever exist? by Maria Papagiannidou-Sen Pier

17-Ten Lies About Aids by Etienne De Harven and Jean-Claude Roussez

18-Mortal Secrets: Truth and Lies in the Age of AIDS by Robert Klitzman and Ronald Bayer

19-Meddling with Mythology: AIDS and the Social Construction of Knowledge by Rosaline S. Barbour and Guro Huby

20-Silence = Death: The Infectious Lie of HIV/AIDS by Niles Stanley

21-When facts lie: A Pragmatics Analysis of the Language Used in Fighting HIV/AIDS in Kenya by Mwangi Gachara

22-AIDS exposed: Secrets,lies & myths:plus the latest breakthrough alternative therapies for AIDS and cancer from rife to ozone

23-The Closing Argument by Charles Ortleb

24-Living Hell: The Truth about AIDS and HIV by Josefina Guardia

25-The Truth About AIDS by Patrick Dixon

26-Truth About HIV by Steven Ransom

27-The AIDS Cover-Up?: The Real and Alarming Facts about AIDS by Gene Antonio

28-The Truth About AIDS: Evolution of an Epidemic by Ann Giudici Fettner and William A. Check

29-Mortal Secrets: Truth and Lies in the Age of AIDS by Robert Klitzman and Ronald Bayer

30-Has Time Finally Revealed the Whole Truth About AIDS?:Exposing a Killer…by Sylvester Chambers

There are many websites on the internet that tell you the truth about AIDS,also.

Just type in the words:

HIV,AIDS,LIE in any major search engine and enjoy the truth!Enjoy written proof as well as video proof!

On this website you will find the names of 2.841 people which are doctors and scientists who already found out that AIDS is a big fat deadly global lie and the number is still growing:

http://aras.ab.ca/rethinkers.php

On this website are 109 Questions for all the "HIV/AIDS" experts:

http://www.areyoupositive.org/gallo.htm

After World War 2 a private company conducted some experiments to see how contagious S.T.D.'s are. They took a group of women that had "S.T.D.'s" and had them have unprotected sex with men that were "S.T.D." free and the other way around. The results were conclusive:The men and women that had S.T.D.'s could not infect the men and women that were "S.T.D." free.

If you are wondering why they never published these historical findings in any magazine or newspaper,don't. They make billions of dollars from these scams called "S.T.D.'s".They don't want people to know the truth and stop making their fortune year after year until one day when the whole world finds out the truth about S.T.D'.s and then they'll be making nothing! Not good for business,eh mate? Bollocks!

There is nothing to fear **here**.

Now **hear** this:

"Fear sells until you stop buying"

Fact:

"All S.T.D.'s are fairy tales"

Do you believe in fairy tales? Then too bad for you! This bullshit definition:

"STD"=Sexually Transmitted Disease"

· is a double lie because of the following 2 reasons:

1)Diseases are NOT contagious meaning NOBODY can give you their disease including an S.T.D.

2)Diseases are NOT caused by bacteria or viruses. According to the scammers S.T.D.'s are "diseases caused by bacteria and viruses".All this means only one thing:

S.T.D.'s do NOT exist.

If I gave you one reason why S.T.D.'s are SCAMS,that would have been good enough but I gave two reasons why S.T.D.'s are SCAMS. Long live free love!

Well,life is full of surprises and I believe this is one of the most shocking pleasant surprises you have ever experienced in your entire life. I know that some of you readers are not gonna believe me and you don't have to believe me or them but believe ONLY the proof behind a story because proof separates a story that is true from a story that is false.

"If you believe that a story is 100% true and that story is 100% false,then I can tell you with 100% certainty that you will suffer the consequences which could be very bad or even deadly"

Here is a real life example:About 15 years ago,7 people were told that they are HIV positive and when they heard these "very bad" news,they all committed suicide. They killed themselves for nothing so be very careful about believing stories without proof.

I know what you are thinking now:if diseases are not contagious and you cannot get an "S.T.D" from having unprotected sex with another person,then what about all those pictures of people that supposedly have STD like symptoms?Let's take herpes for example:people who are "infected" by the herpes virus have lesions, red spots, bumps,blisters and sores on their genitals. Are they proof that the herpes virus causes all that? Absolutely not.

The pictures are real of real people but they are NOT caused by the herpes virus. Remember that viruses don't exist. Herpes genitalis or Herpes is another globally successful SCAM. Some scumbags are making billions of dollars in profit selling you poison(pills) to keep the genital breakouts from reoccuring.

So what's causing all those breakouts on the genitals of men and women? And the breakouts on the lips of people? Toxins.

Fact:

"Any skin breakouts on any part of your body mean only one thing: your body is too toxic"

Virtually everybody is toxic and when the body has too many toxins to eliminate,the body will choose the part of the body where the toxins will be eliminated. For example,when the body eliminates toxins through the nose,it's called a runny nose, when it eliminates extra toxins through the lungs it's called coughing,when it eliminates extra toxins through the face it's called acne,etc. Same thing is happening here:when the body

decides to eliminate the extra toxins through its genitals they call it mistakenly herpes because they say that the herpes virus is causing the outbreaks. Here is another major health secret I'm gonna tell you:Any skin outbreak you have,on any part of your body,it only means one thing:Your body is too toxic and you need to detoxify your body ASAP. So if you are having unprotected sex and after a while you develop some outbreaks on your genitals,that is not proof that your sexual partner gave you an S.T.D. S.T.D.'s don't exist but toxins do. The outbreaks on your genitals were caused by your own body because your body did an emergency toxin elimination. I will explain that in more detail.
Your body is eliminating toxins 24/7:when you sleep and when you are awake to keep itself pure and healthy. You know how you take a shower every day to keep your body pure and healthy on the outside? The body needs to be pure on the inside also to keep itself healthy. In a perfect world,the body can handle eliminating the toxins easily through the 3 organs that eliminate toxins:the skin,the liver and the kidneys and through feces and urine. However,we live in an imperfect world meaning a toxic world:the air we breathe is toxic,the food we eat is toxic and the water we drink is toxic. To make matters worse,stress make our bodies toxic also. When you are having sex,the body uses a lot of its limited energy to give you an orgasm,energy that can be used to eliminate toxins. So,when the body cannot eliminate the toxins of the body because of sex or many other reasons,the body will do an emergency elimination of the toxins which means that the toxins will be eliminated through the skin. I'm gonna expose now another lie:"Some bacteria is bad"

Fact:
"All bacteria is good"

We have billions of bacteria living in our bodies. Without bacteria we would be dead. Bacteria have only one function:to eat the toxins or the garbage in the body. When the body has too many toxins then more bacteria is needed to clean up the body and keep it pure and healthy.
However,that comes with a side-effect:
Extra toxins
Bacteria itself reproduces and produces its own toxins and now you have more toxins in the body.
You might ask,what causes the body to be overloaded with toxins? Simple! We live in a toxic world.
Toxic air,toxic food,toxic water and toxic people!
So,if you ever go and get tested for S.T.D.'s even if you do or you don't have any type of breakouts on your genitals and they tell you that you have one of the following S.T.D.'s:

(About 100 years ago the word virus meant poison)
What you have here is not a disease you got from having unprotected sex with someone,but you have too many toxins in the body and with too many toxins you will have too many bacteria in the body. Bacteria feeds on the toxins of your body and once the food is gone(the toxins and the dead cells of your body),
the bacteria is gone too. Keep your body pure and you will never have to worry a bacterial infection ever again. If your body is pure on the inside,you will never get any breakouts on your genitals after having sex or even when you are not having sex. My priceless advise to you:
Do not even bother to go get tested for S.T.D.'s because you are wasting your precious time and money plus you will be lied to.

Now I would like to expose another old global lie:
FICTION:"Safe sex is having sex with a condom".
This is a bunch of "condomania".
Fact:
"Safe sex is sex WITHOUT a condom"
How much money do you think the condom companies
are making? More than you can imagine!
Business is booming for them!
The truth is exactly the opposite.
Fact:
**"Safe sex is sex without a condom because condoms
are dangerous to you health"**
Their ingredients are highly toxic dangerous chemicals
that can cause birth defects and many other health
problems. Remember "free love" from the 60's when
people were having sex without a condom?They told us
those times are over but I tell you the good times are not
over and they never will be. Free love is alive and well
and party on by getting it on!Enjoy the number one
pleasure in the universe for as long as you want,with as
many people as you want and never worry again about
this global scary deadly lie:
FICTION:
"Sex can give you many diseases or sex can kill you"
Fact:
. **"Sex will never kill you or give you any diseases but
sex will make you feel good and sex is good for your
health,too!Enjoy it for the rest of your life without
any worries whatsoever"**
Remember that saying:"The truth shalt set you free"?
Now that you know the truth feel free to feel good
without any consequences.

Be open-minded and do not ever fear S.T.D.'s ever again. Something that doesn't exist cannot hurt you in any way,shape or form.

Here's more proof that S.T.D.'s don't exist.

I'll end this with the ultimate proof that AIDS is the most evil scam of the 20th century:If you ever get tested for AIDS and the paper comes back positive meaning that you have been "infected" with the HIV virus,relax because the test itself is a fraud and that paper that says you are HIV positive doesn't mean you have the HIV virus. You can have something that does NOT exist.

Fact:

"All HIV tests are false"

They are all scams and they do not detect something that doesn't exist:The HIV virus.

The internet has a lot of videos that prove HIV tests are scams. Go and see for yourself if you want.

I strongly suggest you don't EVER get tested for the HIV virus aka for something that doesn't exist but if you do or if you did,here's what you need to do with the "HIV positive" test paper: Use to wipe your ass with it when you run out of TP for your bunghole!

I have many friends who had "unprotected" sex meaning sex without a condom with hundreds of escorts,swingers,hookers,porn stars and nymphos for more than 30 years and they never got no AIDS,Herpes, Hepatitis or any other nonexistent bullshit "S.T.D."

How is that "posse-ball"? (possible!)

There is only one "sex-plan-ation":

"S.T.D.'s DO NOT EXIST"

They never did and never will.

Check this out,also:I have a lot of male and female friends in the adult industry and every time they get tested for "S.T.D.'s",they only get tested for 3 phoney baloney "S.T.D.'s":1-HIV 2-Chlamydia 3-Gonorrhea What about the other "S.T.D.'s" like herpes, syphilis,hepatitis C,etc? If they really existed then all the adult actors would be infested with them,right? Right,if they existed but fortunately because they don't exist,all my adult movie star male and female friends and all the adult stars in the world have nothing to worry about. Even the 3 tests they get tested for:HIV,Chlamydia and Gonorrhea are a waste of time and money but they are making many companies a lot of money,aren't they? We live in a money hungry world where:

"Money talks and bullshit walks"

Never in my life I heard this from any of my male and female adult movie star friends:I got herpes or I got syphilis or I got Hepatitis C and I never will hear it because you can't get something that doesn't exist.

Show me the conclusive proof of something I know conclusively it doesn't exist! Your honor,I rest my case! If you thought that was impressive,the fact that S.T.D.'s are scams,then check this out:There are a lot more scams out there that could seriously hurt your happiness and I'm gonna expose them all.

FICTION:

"Colds and flus are contagious"

MORE FICTION:

"Colds and flus are caused by bacteria,viruses and cold weather"

Fact:

"Colds are NOT contagious and they are NOT caused by bugs,bacteria,viruses or cold weather"

Babies have 8 colds a year and their parents get colds only once or twice? Where is the contagion here? How is it possible that a man who worked on an observation post in Antarctica "caught" four colds a year? Where did he get the cold from? There was nobody around him! Maybe he got it from Chupacabra! And no,he DID NOT get the cold from the cold weather.

Fact:
"A cold is NOT something you get from anything or anybody"

A few decades ago certain private institutes conducted experiments in the great cold laboratories. In those experiments volunteers were swabbed daily with the cold "viruses" from people that had colds. None of the people swabbed developed a cold,proof positive that colds are NOT contagious.

Do you wanna know the truth about what a cold really is? I'm not gonna be a cold blooded bastard,so I'll tell you!

A cold is the body's emergency way of disposing of too much body waste that it couldn't dispose of through the ordinary channels of elimination.

That's it. It's that simple.

Why have they been lying to us for more than a hundred years? Because telling the people the truth will hurt them big time.

There is a saying:"The truth hurts".In this case the hospitals,the doctors and many other companies that sell cold remedies will be hurt financially in a major way.

They will lose billions of dollars in sales. I never get colds because my body is clean and well nourished and you can be like me:Live cold free!

PS: More than 20 years ago I used to get 4 colds a year and now I get no colds ever!

Here is some proof that colds are not contagious:
1-www.drbass.com
2-http://purewisdom.com.au/colds-no-more-contagious-than-a-bad-mood/
Fact#1:
"Colds and flus are not caused by bacteria or viruses"
Fact#2:
"Colds and flus are NOT contagious"
Fact#3:
"There is a cure for colds and flus"
Fact#4:
"You can live a life without colds and flus"
How? Email me and I'll tell you "the cure" for colds and flus and how to never get a cold or flu again!
So,even the common colds are not contagious. That's shocking but here's something even more shocking:
The "uncommon" cold is not contagious either!
There is no uncommon cold of course but I couldn't help myself but joke again! Common,uncommon-get it?
Come on...Common!
However,what I am about to tell you next is no joke and it can save your life or save you from some major unnecessary suffering.
Fact#5:
"Flu shots are a deadly global scam"
Fact#6:
"Flu shots DO NOT prevent the flu,they cause it"
Getting a flu shot means only one thing:You are poisoning your body with the worst poisons that should never enter a human body like:
Thimerosal,Mercury,Aluminum,Triton x-100,Phenol Ethylene Glycol,Betapropiolactone,Nonoxynol,Octoxinol 9,Sodium Phosphate,Formaldehyde,Sodium

Deoxycholate,MSG (Monosodium Glucamate),
Hydrolyzed porcine gelatin,Gentamicin sulfate,Etc
WARNING:Never ever get the flu shot-it's deadly
2-**FICTION**:Diseases are contagious
So,what have we learned so far?
Germs and viruses don't exist,they don't cause disease
and they are not contagious and bacteria do exist but they
do not cause disease and they are not contagious.
What does all this mean? How the hell should I know?
Wait,I'm the one writing this book so I should know!
To know or "nut" to know! Well,if diseases are NOT
caused by germs,bacteria and viruses,then they are NOT
contagious,either! Make sense?
**"Diseases are NOT contagious and nobody will ever
give you their disease and vice-versa: You cannot give
your own disease to anybody,ever."**
Contagion is one of the oldest and of the most convincing
false stories ever told.
Fact:
"Contagion is a myth"
Diseases are not contagious but lies are. If anybody tells
you that diseases are contagious,they are lying to you just
like somebody else lied to them.
Contagion was born from demonology. Hundreds of
years ago the definition of disease was:You are possessed
by demons. Demons have progressed to evil spirits,to
germs and to bacteria and now to viruses. Fiction is fun!
If diseases were contagious how come we don't catch
heart disease,cancer,asthma, Alzheimer's,Lou Gehrig's
disease,high blood pressure,diabetes,
Parkinson's and so on? So,they are telling us that diseases
come from outside the body. Not true. Cough,cough!
Excuse me but I am allergic to bullshit!

Fact:
"Diseases do not come from outside the body, diseases come from inside the body. Diseases are created by the body. Diseases are body conducted emergency crises of detoxification and healing"

Let me explain that in more detail. The body eliminates toxins from inside that are created by the cells of the body and toxins that get into the body from the bad foods we eat and the bad beverages we drink.

All these inside and outside toxins are eliminated by the body through the 5 organs of elimination I mentioned earlier. Unfortunately, 99% of the world's population is toxic meaning they have too many toxins in the body.

So, what happens when the body has too many toxins to eliminate? It creates what is called "disease".

Contrary to popular belief, disease is something good not something bad. Disease is the emergency removal of extra toxins so the body can keep itself healthy.

If disease didn't exist then we would drop dead when the body is too toxic. When the 5 organs of elimination cannot cope with the task of keeping the body clean, then a crisis or emergency called sickness or disease is initiated so the body can do its job which is cleansing and repairing itself.

Here is another tremendous health secret I'm gonna tell you right now:

"There were never any cures for any diseases and there never will be"

No doctor and no remedy can cure you from any disease. Introducing another mind blowing health secret:

"The disease itself is the cure"

And they are trying to cure diseases! Talk about pure stupidity! Pure idiocy! Pure nonsense! Pure bullshit!

You get my message,right mate? Crikey mate!
Guess who can cure the body?

Fact:

"Only the body can cure itself"

Here's an example:Let's say you are riding a skateboard too fast and accidentally you fall off it and break your a few bones and cut you skin in many places. Does any doctor or remedy cure you? No!

"The body cures itself if given the proper care"

You don't need to do anything except wear a cast and some bandages and wait. The body is very intelligent and continuously repairs itself and there's almost nothing the body cannot repair.

Fact:

"There is no such thing as an incurable disease"

All diseases are curable and your body will do the job if given the right tools which are in many cases supplements,natural treatments,rest,etc.

Diseases are caused by the condition of the body of the patient. In 1914 a series of experiments were conducted in which the germs that supposedly cause hay fever, dyphteria, pneumonia,tuberculosis, meningitis,etc were added to the food and drinks of a group of volunteers.

The results were:No volunteer got sick. Almost everybody believes that germs are transmitted from one person to another but this experiment is proof positive that diseases are not contagious.

Remember that there is no contagious disease only contagious habits that make you sick. A group of people that had dyphteria were studied and no germ was found in them to blame for the disease. The same thing can be said about tuberculosis and other diseases.

That's why the virus was invented to save the theory:"Germs cause disease".Now we have infections caused by viruses instead of germs because the pathologists couldn't find a single germ for all human diseases. If a germ doesn't cause disease then what causes it? Soon mankind will learn that the lifestyle of an individual causes disease. Stress,your diet and your drinks cause disease. A healthy child could sleep in the same bed with a child "infected" by chicken pox,scarlet fever,mumps,measles or any other "infectious disease" and will never be infected by any disease.

Not everybody on this planet believes that diseases are contagious. All natural hygienists know that diseases are not contagious.

There is a science called Natural Hygiene and anybody who practices it,it's called a Natural Hygienist. See for yourself. Here you will find a few doctors that practice natural hygiene:

http://naturalhygienesociety.org/doctors.html

Contact them and ask them and if diseases are contagious and see what they say. And if any of them say diseases are contagious,then tell them that they are fired!

Also,tell them that:

Their eyes are brown because they are full of shit! Contagion is just an old global lie that is making many companies billions of dollars in profit. Imagine how much money they would lose if people knew the truth? Too much money to mention here!

And in this case it hurts the rich evil greedy ones financially. We are talking a loss of billions upon billions of dollars here,people. The evil greedy rich bastards wanna stay rich,even if they have to lie to the entire planet.

The rich-the greedy evil ones-only care about two things:

1-Keep up their profits

2-Make more profits

They never cared about the poor and they never will.
Or will they? Some day?
Time will tell but it might take some time until that happens. Or it might never happen.
They also tell us that they are so close to finding a cure for certain diseases and that is yet again another big skinny lie! (big fat lie).
They never found a cure for a single disease out there and they never will.
By the way:If you think they cured polio with a vaccine then think again:They didn't cure anything.
Polio was a scam born in the 40's and it made some serious money for the bad guys.
Here's some proof that:

POLIO was a major SCAM

1)http://www.thebirdman.org/Index/Others/Others-Doc-Health&Medicine/+Doc-Health&Medicine-MscCures&Suggestions/PolioCausedByPoisons_files/current16.htm

2)http://gdsajj.wordpress.com/tag/polio-vaccine-scam/

3)http://vaccineresistancemovement.org/?p=814

They-the compulsive lying bastards-also tell us that:
1-Colds have no cure and they are contagious
2-Colds are caused by bugs,germs,bacteria,viruses and cold weather
You probably should now by now that once again all these stories are for gullible people!More lies my esteemed colleagues.

More lies=More money

WARNING: Your medical doctor is dangerous to your health or even deadly and he doesn't have perfect health and he will never teach you how to have and enjoy perfect health forever.

Also,he will tell you many times nasty things you never wanna hear,like:

1-I don't know the cause of this or that disease

2-I don't know the cure for such and such disease

3-You have 6 months to 9 months live,etc

Exception:There are some medical doctors out there that are actually smart!

Here are some very important things you'll never hear from your poorly educated medical doctor.

Doctors are richly educated in treating your symptoms with drugs and surgery which are both barbaric,inhumane and many times deadly treatments.

Fire your MD or you'll have to answer to me!

The body,while complex by design,is very simple in operation. When you take drugs,eat bad food like meat,cooked food,etc,drink, smoke,vaccinate your body repeatedly and stifle your symptoms with medications then your body has no choice but to find a way to get rid of all this toxic stuff you've been dumping into it.

So,when your body can't take the abuse anymore,it forces a detoxification to eliminate all of the toxins you have been ingesting.

You think that disease is something bad because that's what they told you but they lied to you.

Disease is good for you because:

Fact:

"Disease is your body's way of making you healthier"

Your medical doctor will give you:

"A pill for every ill"

Fact:
"Pills or prescribed drugs are deadly chemicals and should never ever be ingested"

That applies to prescribed pills and OTC pills also.
(OTC=Over-The-Counter)
Pills kill millions of people around the world every day. They are literally chemicals or poisons and they should never ever be taken because they cause disease,suffering and death.

"The best medicine is no medicine"

Here is some wise advise from a very wise man from a long time ago:

"Nearly all men die of their medicines,not of their diseases."

Did this guy know something we don't know today? Yes he did and now you know too!

By taking in toxins,you kill your cells and when you destroy cells,bacteria are attracted to these diseased areas. Then you go to your medical doctor and he finds bacteria. He immediately assumes you have a bacterial infection and you are sick. And the bacteria made you sick. Not true at all. Your medical doctor just blew smoke up your ass! Or in other words,he or she lied to you.

Fact:
"Most diseases are actually body-initiated detoxifications for the purpose to bring back balance to the body or to keep the body clean or free of toxins"

That's why diseases are good for you!Just like you need to have your room clean so you can walk around in it,the body needs to be clean also,so it can function properly. If you would stop taking the trash from the kitchen for example,what would happen after a while?

The kitchen would be so full of trash that you couldn't enter it anymore. The kitchen would become a landfill or a trash storage room. So the kitchen is no longer your kitchen where you enjoy your food every day. Same thing happens with your body:you are no longer gonna enjoy perfect health if your body is dirty on the inside,get it?

Now that you got it,what are you gonna do with it? The more the body is forced to store toxic substances within its cells,joints,tissues,organs and bones,the more the health of the body degrades and the closer you are getting to aging and dying.

"Health is created only by healthy living"

Our bodies are miraculous. They have the capacity to self direct,to self construct,self protect,self preserve,self maintain and self repair. Our bodies are perfect and they act perfectly all the time. The human body has his own system that rebuilds,purifies and heals. For example,if we cut our finger accidentally,all we have to do is put a band-aid on it and wait. The body does the healing.

We create all our health problems that make us suffer except of course for the people that are born with health problems already. We are our own enemies.

We are making ourselves sick

Here is another major life changing health secret:

"The only cure for disease is the disease itself"

When the body detoxifies,it is in the process of curing or healing itself and any interference of this process spells disaster. All medications serve to suppress symptoms. All of them are neurotransmitter inhibitors or accelerators capable of tampering with the proper neurological functioning of the body. Tampering with this function causes malfunction within the body. Cells are forced to operate in ways they wouldn't normally operate,the nervous system is forced to shut down and the body is damaged severely. Liquid-releasing symptoms are suppressed for purposes of curing the disease and the medical doctors never realize that these symptoms are the body's way of healing itself. All medications are toxic to cells. All medications, including vaccinations and antibiotics,are toxic to the body and are destroying the body from the inside out.

"Educate,don't medicate"

Children who are taking prescribed drugs could develop these nasty side-effects:tics,mania,liver failure,allergies,psychosis,convulsions, psychosis, cellular damage,joint and cartilage deterioration,etc. Psychoactive(drugs for the brain)drugs such as are responsible for causing more serious side-effects like:bouts of depression,some so severe they have led users to murder their families and kill themselves.

Fact:

"In America,over 250,000 people each year die of prescription medications they were told to take by their medical doctors and they were taking the drugs the way they were supposed to be taken. Around the world prescribed drugs kill millions of people"

Drugs,whether illegal, prescription or over-the-counter, are dangerous and deadly to the human body and to the overall health and wellness of anyone who takes them.

Remember the slogan against illegal drugs:

"Don't do drugs"

Here's my version of that:

Don't do prescribed or over-the-counter drugs because they are gonna do you in....inside a coffin!

Here's another major global deadly scam:
VACCINES
FICTION:
"Vaccines prevent disease"
and
MORE FICTION:
"Vaccines eliminated a lot of diseases"
Fact:
"Vaccines cause disease and death. Vaccines cause autism,paralysis,etc. Never ever vaccinate yourself because if you do the consequences are devastating"
Here's another deadly global lie against our pets:
FICTION:
"Vaccinate your pets against rabies"
Fact:
"Rabies is a scam"
it doesn't exist so if you love your pets never ever give them any vaccines. The ingredients in almost all vaccines are the deadliest poisons you can ever imagine like:
Formaldehyde,Aspartame,Mercury,Mono-sodium glutamate (MSG),Phosphate,Bacterial Waste, Aluminum potassium sulfate,Aluminum,Antibiotics, Hydroxyde, Thimerosal,Glycerin,Phenol, Sorbitol, Phenoxyethenol, Cancerous Cells,Feces,Urine,etc.
Yuck,that's gross and disgusting.
I call that:"Dis-gross-ting"!
WARNING:Do not ever vaccinate yourself,your kids or your pets,EVER.
Fact #1:
"Vaccines cause disease,they don't prevent it"
Fact#2:
"Vaccines cause many horrible diseases and death"

Diseases like measles,mumps,chicken pox,etc. But what did they tell us about the above diseases? They told us that those diseases have disappeared thanks to vaccines. So they are telling us that vaccines cure diseases. Really? I'm not convinced!

FICTION:

"The tragic truth is that no vaccine has ever eradicated any disease and no vaccine ever will"

These evil bastards are monsters. They tell us these deadly evil lies who destroy families and make millions of innocent people suffer needlessly and die.

Who cares about the people,right? As long as these greedy evil heartless soulless demons make billions of dollars in profit.

Vaccines also cause other horrible diseases like:diabetes, lung cancer,epilepsy,polio, asthma,rubella,brain damage, nervous system malfunction, anaphylactic shock(extreme allergic reaction),arthritis, Alzheimer's disease,cancer,etc.

It gets worse:vaccines also killed millions of babies worldwide and unfortunately it's still happening today. When babies would die from Shaken baby syndrome they blamed it on many innocent parents who were arrested and charged with the crime of killing their newborn children in violent attempts to get them to stop crying and go back to sleep. When babies died of crib death-also known as sudden infant death syndrome or SIDS,they couldn't blame that on anybody or anything because they didn't know what killed these precious poor newborn babies.

Now educated people like me and you know the real cause for The shaken baby syndrome and SIDS:(Sudden Infant Death Syndrome):Vaccines

Vaccines:they are the cause for the baby genocide. Here's how this deadly evil scam works: According to them inoculations or vaccinations work on the premise that our bodies will create antibodies to the pathogens (deadly toxins) found within the vaccines. If we have antibodies,we are immune to the particular disease in question. If we are immune,we can't catch disease. This theory of theirs sounds very convincing but what about AIDS? With most other diseases,if you have the antibodies to that disease,you cannot catch the disease because you are immune to the disease but with AIDS,if you have the antibodies to HIV, you are said to be HIV-positive and at risk for AIDS.

This is also the case with all other "viral" diseases. Since no one can find a virus (which is a blatant violation of Koch's postulates,one of the cornerstones of the contagion theory),the only way to detect a virus is to detect its antibodies. But if we have antibodies,we're immune!That's the whole premise of immunization. So,on the one hand,if you have antibodies,you have immunity but on the other hand,if you have antibodies you are at risk. These murderous idiots are contradicting themselves. They tell us two contradicting stories and they tell us they are both true stories. That's like saying:The milk is white-true story. The milk is black-also true story. They may have fooled virtually everybody on this planet but not me. And you my precious reader now know the truth and they can't fool you anymore.

Even more important,they cannot poison you legally and make you really sick or worse:kill you with their deadly legal poison they call:Vaccines

Fact:
Vaccinated=Terminated
To get vaccinated means to poison your blood which means expect disease,suffering and premature death. Again,the body is very simple in operation. If you drink or eat something that it cannot use,your body immediately tries to get rid of it. The more toxins you give your body,the more your body tries to eliminate them but there comes a time when these toxins are stored in the cells of your body for too long.

The normal channels of elimination such as defecation,urination, respiration and perspiration are enough to eliminate all toxic substances from the body but when toxins are stored for prolonged periods of time,they must be eliminated through alternate channels and that is why you develop symptoms such as irritability,fatigue,drowsiness,nausea,diarrhea, constipation,vomiting,bloating,fever,headaches,trouble sleeping,nightmares,nasal drip,coughing, sneezing, pustules,boils,skin breakouts,acne,congestion,flu like symptoms,pain,etc.

Detoxify or die
And it's not gonna be a quick painless death. It's gonna be a long(years or decades) slow agonizing painful death. Your body uses these alternate channels for the purposes of detoxification but according to them,what are you supposed to do when you develop such symptoms? You are supposed to take medications(more toxins)to relieve yourself of these symptoms. How moronic!

So if you listen to them,you stop the detoxification, which forces your body to restore the toxins,thus setting you up for a more difficult detoxification in the future

and if you never detoxify your body,then expect some major suffering in your future or an early death.
If you want perfect health,then you better do the perfect detox which is a yearly detox!
Lately,they came up with more scams than ever:
The flu shot
The swine flu
The avian flu
The H1N1 flu
The H3N4 flu
The West Nile Virus
SARS
Legionnaire's disease
Lyme disease
Whopping cough(TDAP)
Shingles,Etc
"They lie so you can buy"
But I tell you not to buy....this lie!
In the future they will come up with more scams because the more scams they come up with the more money they make. **Do not believe** these evil deadly lies because they could make you **very sick or kill you.**
I hope you enjoyed reading my book and I hope you enjoyed my sense of humor! For those of you who didn't enjoy my sense of humor,I have 2 messages for you:
1-You dropped something..............................your smile!
2-You dropped something else........your sense of humor!
PS:If you don't have a sense of humor,buy one!
Sometimes the truth hurts (only if you are closed-minded) but in reality the truth NEVER hurts.
The truth never hurts me. It never did and never will.
Let's see now what other intelligent people have said about the truth!

"All truth goes through three stages.
1-First it is ridiculed.
2-Then it is violently opposed.
3-Finally,it is accepted as self-evident"
Arthur Schopenhauer

"A lie can travel half way around the world while the truth is putting on its shoes"
Mark Twain

"Never tell the truth to people who are not worthy of it"
Mark Twain

"The truth is rarely pure and never simple"
Oscar Wilde

"The truth will set you free, but first it will piss you off"
Gloria Steinem

"When I despair, I remember that all through history the way of truth and love have always won. There have been tyrants and murderers, and for a time, they can seem invincible, but in the end, they always fall. Think of it--always"
Mahatma Gandhi

"Facts do not cease to exist because they are ignored"
Aldous Huxley

"It's not hard to find the truth. What is hard is not to run away from it once you have found it"
Prometheus

"All truths are easy to understand once they are discovered;the point is to discover them"
Galileo Galilei

"Tell the truth, or someone will tell it for you"
Stephanie Klein

I did my job,I told you the truth! Happy now?
I hope you enjoyed reading my unique life changing book and if you have any comments,questions or suggestions please email me. Thank you very much and I wish you a delicious sex life free from worry. You no longer have to fear these LIES/SCAMS called S.T.D.'s!
Happy care free orgasms!
Tony Davis,P.H.T.
Perfect Health Teacher
Email:SicaBulex@Gmail.com
Http://www.HappyForever.us

www.ingramcontent.com/pod-product-compliance
Lightning Source LLC
Chambersburg PA
CBHW070326290526
45791CB00003B/1271